# NATURAL RECIPES TO STRENGTHEN THE IMMUNE SYSTEM AND BEAT THE CURRENT DISEASE

Health & Wellness

# NATURAL RECIPES TO STRENGTHEN THE IMMUNE SYSTEM AND BEAT THE CURRENT DISEASE

BY **SILVIA ALVAREZ**

**JUNE 2020**

First Edition: June 2020
KDP ISBN No. 9798655976955
Edited by Silvia Alvarez
Copyright © 2020. Silvia Alvarez.
Printed in Peru
No part of this work can be reproduced by any means without the Author's permission.
The ink we use is chlorine free and the inner paper type is acid free.
Both products are supplied by a supplier certified by the Forest Stewardship Council (FSC Forest Stewarchip) The paper is made with 30% recycled waste material.

# INDEX

INTRODUCTION
CHAPTER 1
Immune system:
 Natural recipes to increase defenses:
 Vitamins and minerals to increase defenses:.
Recommendations to Strengthen the Immune System:
Foods that stimulate your Immune System and Strengthen Defenses
CHAPTER 2
NATURAL RECIPES
TO FIGHT COVID19 AND STRENGTHEN THE IMMUNE SYSTEM:
Tea No. 2 to Cure the Virus or Flu:
Tea No. 3 to Cure and Prevent Covid 19:
Syrup to fight viruses and flu:
Tea to Increase the Body's Defenses: (Very Effective):
Recipes to fight Respiratory Infections, Flu, Asthma, Covid19, strengthen the Immune System.
Recipe No. 2. to raise the Defenses:
Recipe No. 3. to raise the Defenses:
Recipe No. 4. to strengthen the Defenses:
Recipe No. 5. to raise the Defenses:
Recipe No. 6. to increase Defenses and combat Covid19:
Recipe No. 7. Seville Lemon Water, to increase the Defenses quickly:
Recipe No. 8. To increase defenses very quickly:
Recipe No. 8. Shot of Ginger and Turmeric to raise the defenses:
Vegetable Salad Recipe to Strengthen Defenses:

# BIBLIOGRAPHY

- Consultation Dr. Elmer Vilchez
- El Universal newspaper.
- El Español newspaper
- Consultation Dr. Franklin Suárez
- Rossio de Jesús Rodríguez Lobo (Inhabitant of Pucallpa, Peru)

# INTRODUCTION

The presence of the Covid-19 virus pandemic in the world has caused many scientists to carry out research to counteract the presence of this virus and others that may appear in the future, and has made us meditate each of us seriously, how we could overcome and stay healthy from this and any other disease. Viruses attack weakened organisms, organisms with one or more diseases. Diseases are the product of a weak immune system, therefore, through food we generate good or bad nutrition that helps us defend our good health.

Without a specific treatment, and without a vaccine that is expected in the near horizon, the only defense that our body has against Covid-19 is our Immune systems, how our immune system responds to infection will depend on the results, we can suffer from symptoms mild like dry cough, sore throat, tiredness, fever, severe symptoms like pneumonia, acute respiratory problems until failure multi-organic and death.

The immune system is a complex network of cells, organs and tissues that work together to defend ourselves against microorganisms and toxic substances that are present in the world around us and that could make us sick. Experts have explained in numerous articles how to strengthen this system to better face Covid-19 and all diseases in general, recommending a healthy diet, sleep, avoid stress, avoid alcohol, tobacco and other toxic substances. The importance of knowing what we eat has to do with the substances found in food that allows us to strengthen our immune system. The consumption of foods rich in arginine has always been recommended, which is important for the production of collagen and generates scarring if an injury is found at the level of mucus or the respiratory tract.

It should be noted that the foods in the recipes that I am providing through this book such as lemon, garlic, ginger and onion are powerful foods that strengthen our immune system. Here I also offer the recipe with which they are fighting covid19 in Peru, (Chapter 2, Tea No. 3), which they can prepare in case they contract the virus, they can even prepare it without being sick to be stronger and overcome quickly this sickness.

# CHAPTER 1

Next we explain how the Immune system works and then we will see how to strengthen it, explaining in detail the recipes and recommendations to upload and keep our Immune system in perfect working order

**Immune system:**

It is a group of cells, tissues and organs with special tasks for the protection of the human body. The cells that make up the immune system develop from main stem cells in the liver and bone marrow and also in lymph nodes, spleen and lymph. The tactic of the immune system authorizes the rapid production of a large number of cells that stop an infection or an attack on the body.

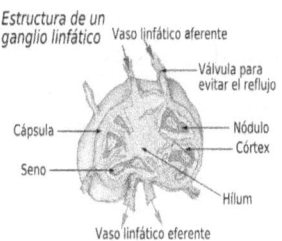

**Function of the Immune system:** The Immune system presents two types of responses to foreign substances. The first, are the natural responses, occur when the infectious focus is found and the immune system reacts immediately, there is no memory of exposure to that focus. The second type is acquired responses, called accommodation, that act when there is repeated exposure to a given infection. The innate response uses phagocyte cells, which trap foreign substances, destroy or transport them, release inflammatory substances, or release natural killer cells.

The immune system defends the body from germs that can invade it such as viruses, bacteria, fungi and parasites that can make us sick. The main cells of the immune system, lymphocytes, can travel through the blood and the lymphatic system, which allows detecting invaders.

In normal situations the immune system has the ability to distinguish between own and foreign cells and tissues, it can remind ancient invaders to develop a specific response to inhibit or destroy them.

**What can affect the Immune system:** An autoimmune disease is a medical condition in which the immune system becomes the aggressor that attacks and destroys the body's own healthy organs and tissues. Normally, the immune system distinguishes the proper from the strange and defends us from external agents such as viruses or bacteria. Certain people are genetically susceptible to developing autoimmune diseases. However, to damage the immune system there are other risk factors involved such as environmental, poor diet, hormones, medications, tobacco.

**Immune system diseases:** Among the diseases that affect the immune system are arthritis, allergies, celiac disease, inflammatory bowel disease. Other diseases that alter the defenses and trigger the immune process are lupus, Sjogren's syndrome, Hashimoto's thyroiditis, type 1 diabetes, Graves' disease. For example, arthritis occurs when the immune system attacks lining tissues and damages the joints. More than 80 autoimmune diseases have been recognized that present signs alike.

## *Natural recipes to increase defenses:*

In the face of the Covid-19 pandemic, many people wonder if it is possible to strengthen their immune system to prevent infection. You should know that it is difficult to get it in a short time, but it is recommended to include foods rich in vitamins A, B, C and E (which can be supplemented with vitamin supplements) and others such as fruits, vegetables or blue fish. It is even advisable decrease the consumption of sugars and ultra-processed foods, perform moderate physical exercise and rest properly.

**How to know if your defenses are low:** Blood tests show the presence of elements harmful to our body and also the lack of certain substances that it produces naturally, but they are not able to show if a person is weak, tired or if his body is especially vulnerable to diseases.

### Vitamins and minerals to increase defenses:

- **Vitamin B:** They form a group of 8 vitamins related to cellular metabolism. These vitamins are found in whole grains, rice, oats, wheat germ, and legumes.

- **Vitamin C:** It helps wound healing, improves the absorption of iron present in food and contributes to the proper functioning of the immune system to protect the body against diseases. Vitamin C is found in: blackcurrant, guava, parsley, red pepper, Brussels sprouts, broccoli, kiwis, papaya, orange, and fennel bulb.

- **Iron:** It is essential in the production of hormones and connective tissues. Its absence can cause anemia. The foods that contain the most iron are lentils, spinach, raspberries, brewer's yeast, pistachios, cereals such as millet and spirulina, a type of blue algae that is attributed with numerous beneficial properties for health.

- **Vitamin D:** helps calcium absorption and is essential for maintaining bone health, improves cellular metabolism, muscle function and defense against infection. Besides the sun, the foods that contain this vitamin are cod liver oil, blue fish, shellfish, liver, dairy, eggs, mushrooms, avocado and wheat germ. Other foods that we can include in our diet are: onion and garlic in all meals. Both are foods that help fight virus and bacteria infections. Garlic must be eaten raw to maintain its properties, while onion does not lose its properties when cooked.

- **Zinc:** It is a component that helps the immune system fight bacteria and viruses that invade the body. The richest foods in zinc are: oysters, beef liver, clams, ,red meat, hazelnuts and almonds, chicken and turkey, cheese and oatmeal.

✓ **Honey:** It is a good substitute for sugar, since it has antioxidant and antibacterial properties that sugar does not have. Finally, Ginger is rich in vitamins, potassium and niacin, and has properties that help fight infections caused by viruses and bacteria. In addition, it has antitussive and expectorant characteristics that fight colds and the flu.

## Probiotics:

They are foods with a high presence of live microorganisms that enhance the activity of the bacterial flora already present in our body and, with this, contribute to the normality of the internal processes of the human body.

1. Kimchi: Like sauerkraut, it is a cabbage fermentation, common in Korean cuisine, very spicy and has great probiotics properties, although it should be avoided when packaged.
2. Dark Chocolate: Fermentation of the cocoa bean, rich in flavonoids, which are highly antioxidants.
3. Natto: Fermentation of soybean paste that provides a high protein content, in addition to vitamin B12. It is not widely used in the West yet, but it is very popular in Southeast Asia.
4. Miso: Fermentation of Koji mushroom and soy beans, it has a strong flavor and provides a large amount of lactobacillus.
5. Pickles: Although they provide an important quantity of beneficial microorganisms their consumption must be punctual, since it is a very acidic food.
6. Kefir: Very similar to yogurt it provides a rich micro bacterial flora, including lactobacillus and bifids.

## *Foods that lower defenses:*

*1.  **Alcohol:*** *Alcohol consumption decreases the production of white blood cells.*

*2.  **Sugars:*** *Sugar consumption has been shown to decrease immune activity for a few hours and therefore momentarily weaken us.*

*3. **Preservatives and additives:*** *Some of the substances used to preserve certain foods are seen by our Immune system as a threat, so the smaller the amount of preservatives, dyes, acidulants, flavor enhancers and other additives that are consumed the less work will be on or immune system.*

*4. **Foods to which you are allergic or intolerant:*** *It is important to detect food allergic and intolerances, even if they are mild problems because they force the immune system to work twice es hard, if one is allergic to lactose, for example, consuming milk will trigger an immune response that would be unnecessary if one were to go carefully and avoid such consumption. Therefore, if you have the slightest suspicion that a particular food does not feel good to you, you should consult the doctor about the matter are soon as possible.*

## *Recommendations to Strengthen the Immune System:*

Keeping us in a state of anxiety and stress, makes our body weak, stimulating the production of cortisol (hydrocortisone) , called the stress hormone, which has a direct and negative influence on our health, Stress and lows They have a similar effect, so, within this Covit-19 crisis, it is necessary to maintain the most positive vision of life, if it can be without chemicals, the better. This type of attitude has enormous advantages for the body: it increases the level of immunoglobulin, which is an antibody, relaxes the muscles and releases endorphins, which, in turn, generates greater well-being.

The following recommendations will allow our immune system to remain healthy and stable:

- **Get enough sleep:** Not getting enough sleep is another of the causes of deterioration of our immunity, since when sleeping, our body recovers from the work done during the day, this is noticeable in our immune system.

- The immune system suffers greatly from the consequences of poor rest habits, and instead benefits from adequate sleep and the necessary hours.

- **Brush your teeth well:** Poor mouth hygiene can affect the function of the immune system, this is because aggressive bacteria are created and proliferate that can alter the body's immune response function, as we age our immune system becomes more sensitive and delicate and As there is poor oral hygiene, the increase in bad bacteria is associated with the development of pneumonia in adults, which is a serious common consequence that is being observed in covid19. We must brush our teeth for a minimum period of two minutes.

- **Exercise and maintain a weight appropriate to your height:** Sedentary lifestyle and being overweight hinder the circulation of blood, as well as the correct oxygenation of our body, it is recommended to exercise constantly at least three times a week.

- **Eliminate sugar:** Consuming sugar increases inflammatory substances in the body, these substances gradually lower the body's defenses that are the key to fighting viruses. One of the reasons that refined sugar affects the immune system is that it has a high glycemic index, which means increased blood sugar, reducing the responsiveness of white blood cells, the lymphocytes that produce antibodies. Antibodies are important because they defend us from viruses and bacteria, expelling them from the body. In addition, the antibodies create memory of the viruses, thus giving us immunity.

- **Eliminate fats in meals:** Diets rich in fats and foods high in sugars: these diets fill our bodies with sugar fats and saturated fats and low nutrients, which increases our weight and increases the harmful substances in our blood, running the risk of lowering our defenses and get diabetes and cardiovascular disease.

- **Avoid consuming** dairy, sugar, cheese, yogurt, as they inflame the organs.

- **Avoid consuming wheat, rice and corn regularly** since they contain gluten, then the Harms of eating these foods continuously:

Intestinal permeability, favors liver diseases, hypothyroidism, asthma, Crohn's disease, seizures, is related to cases of autism and schizophrenia. By reducing the consumption of wheat, rice or corn, blood sugar levels are reduced, there are cases of prediabetics and diabetics that have stopped being it and improvement of various conditions such as: arthritis, psoriasis, chronic sinusitis, intestinal irritation.

- **It is also very important to maintain very careful personal hygiene:** Simply washing your hands prevents the spread of diseases like Covid-19. As the hands touch everything, they become a source of germs that you will eliminate with good hygiene or good hand sanitizer, in the case of being away from home.

## *Foods that stimulate your Immune System and Strengthen Defenses*

You can choose natural remedies, which are available to everyone and have been passed down from generation to generation. If you have a runny nose, fever, or other flu discomfort, you can consume:

- **Tara for a sore throat**: Tare is widely used as an anti-inflammatory to remove pain. You can make an infusion with 6 pods or a tablespoon of ground tare in 2 cups of water. It is recommended to gargle in the morning so that the phlegm does not bother during the day.

- **Fever**: A warm bath with closed doors without drafts can lower the temperature. Using an ice pack is not recommended because it can complicate patients with pneumonia.

- **Infusion of garlic, kion, lemon and honey**: It can improve the Immune system. Garlic contains allicin, a natural anti-inflammatory that regenerates the immune system. Kion or ginger has camphor, a decongestant in upper respiratory processes.

- **Inhalation with eucalyptus leaves**: it is effective against nasal and bronchial congestion.

**Citric fruits:** The most popular way to boost your immune system is to increase the consumption of citrus fruits. Citrus fruits are packed with vitamin C, which helps increase white blood cells (called leukocytes). White blood cells help your body fight infection. Citrus fruits include oranges, grapefruits, lemons, limes, tangerines, and clementines, to name a few.

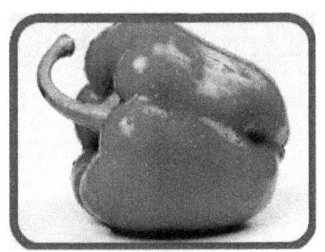

**Red peppers:** Red peppers have more vitamin C than citrus. These delicious vegetables are also an excellent source of beta carotene. This means that eating more red bell peppers during cold and flu season can help strengthen your defenses with its antioxidant properties and keep your eyes healthy with beta carotene.

**Garlic:** I don't know if you like it as much as I do, but garlic is an ingredient that is not lacking in my kitchen. Garlic is famous for fighting infections thanks to its sulfur-containing compounds, such as allicin. It is believed to be the reason 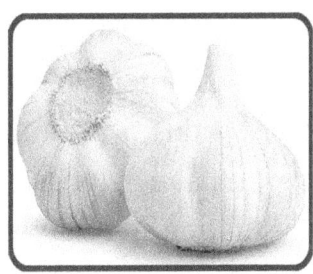 why, even in ancient times, our ancestors used garlic as a means of fighting infections naturally.

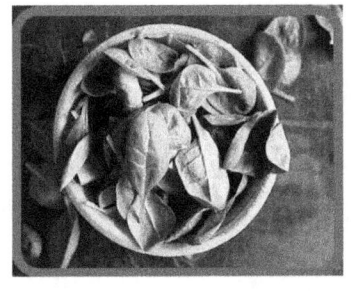

**Spinach:** Spinach is a vegetable very rich in nutrients and super versatile. You can eat raw or cooked spinach, making it a great addition to any favorite salad or recipe. Consider sautéing the spinach in butter and garlic to add to the scrambled eggs for an extra dose of antioxidants. This helps strengthen the immune system during the cold and flu season. You can also add fresh spinach to your morning smoothie.

**Kiwis:** These green fruits are loaded with vitamin C. Kiwis also have vitamin E, K, folic acid and potassium. Another good news? They are an excellent source of fiber.

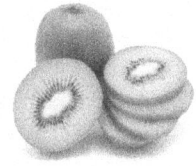

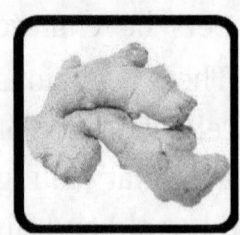

**Ginger:** Known as a powerful natural medicine, ginger fights nausea and has anti-inflammatory properties. This flowering plant can also help fight the common cold.

**Turmeric or stick:** A powerful natural anti-inflammatory, turmeric (and its active compound, curcumin) is packed with antioxidants. This spice can be added to smoothies, juices, and chicken. It also adds a bright orange color. These

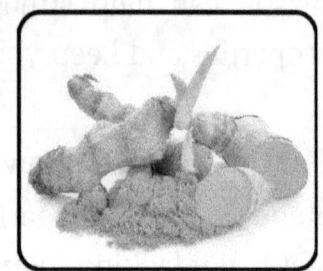

are just some foods that you can add to your daily diet to start stimulating the defenses and the Immune system of all our family. We have no idea when the new covid19 it will stop spreading, for now it is part of our life. I hope that these natural options to strengthen the immune system can help us stay as healthy as possible.

# CHAPTER 2

## Natural Recipes to fight covid 19 the virus and strengthen the Immune System

Covid-19 is probably fatal only for certain risk groups, which are determined based on age and who suffer from preliminary diseases. According to statistics, 81% of cases are mild and overcome the disease without any problem, but it is life threatening in people over 80, with other aliments or low defenses. The immune system is complicate, but it correct functioning is decisive for our body to withstand external attacks, therefore it must be cared for and strengthened as far as possible. I will tell you how to help prevent the spread of covid19 and any other diseases by strengthening the immune system of your body through your diet, prepare the following recipes and you will notice how wonderful theses foods are.

## Tea No. 1 to Cure and Prevent Covid 19:
**Ingredients:**

01 Onion

02 Garlic Cloves

½ lemon

02 Glasses of Water

02 Cinnamon Sticks

**Preparation:** Peel the garlic, and remove the peel from the onions, chop it into 4 pieces, place the water, the lemon juice, bring to a boil with all the ingredients, also place the cinnamon, cover, let it boil for 15 minutes. Then serve hot and take 3 times a day.

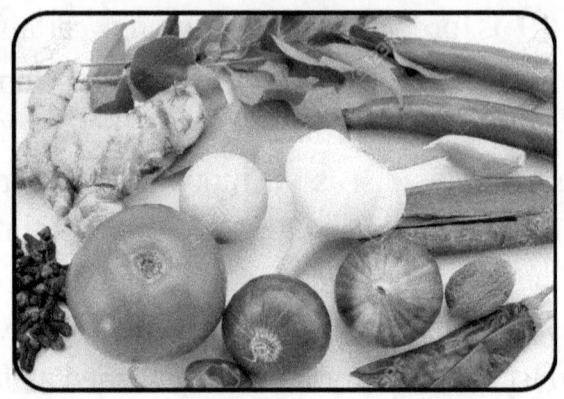

## *Tea No. 2 to Cure the Virus or Flu:*

**Ingredients:**

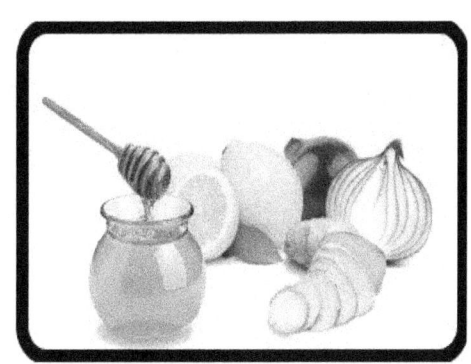

01 red onion, large

01 Garlic Head

02 Ginger Root

03 Pieces of Cinnamon

01 Bunch of Coriander

02 Lemons

02 oranges

02 tablespoons of honey

**Preparation:** In a saucepan place the water, chop the garlic head in 2, and remove the peels from the onions, chop it into 4 pieces, add the lemons and oranges, chop the ginger into small pieces, add the coriander, bring to a boil with All the ingredients, also place the cinnamon, cover, boil for 20 minutes over low heat. Then serve and take 3 times a day.

## *Tea No. 3 to Cure and Prevent Covid 19:*
**Ingredients:**

01 purple onion

03 Garlic Cloves

01 Lemon

02 Glasses of Water

01 Small Ginger Root.

03 Eucalyptus Leaves

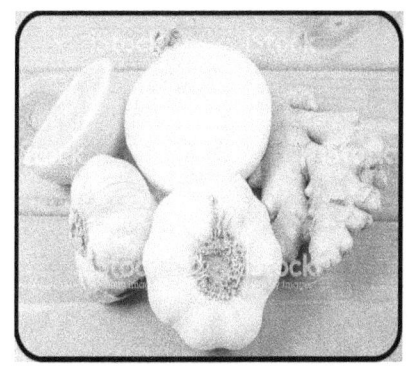

**Preparation:** In a saucepan place the water, chop the garlic, and remove the peels from the onions, chop it into 4 pieces, chop the ginger into small pieces, bring to a boil with all the ingredients, cover, simmer for 10 minutes over low heat. Then serve and add the lemon juice, place the eucalyptus leaves, take 3 times a day.

**Syrup to fight viruses and flu:** *This Syrup is very effective to fight covid19, the flu and strengthen defenses:*

### Ingredients:

02 Centimeters of ginger root

02 large garlic

½ Cup of Honey

½ red onion

**Preparation:** Peel and chop the onions, ginger and garlic, crush them in a mortar, then put it in a glass bottle, add the honey. Let stand 8 to 12 hours.

**Adults:** take 1 tablespoon 2 to 3 times a day, for 7 days, rest and resume in 7 days more approximately. Children older than 3 years: take 1 teaspoon twice a day (morning and night), for 7 days, rest and resume in 7 days more approximately.

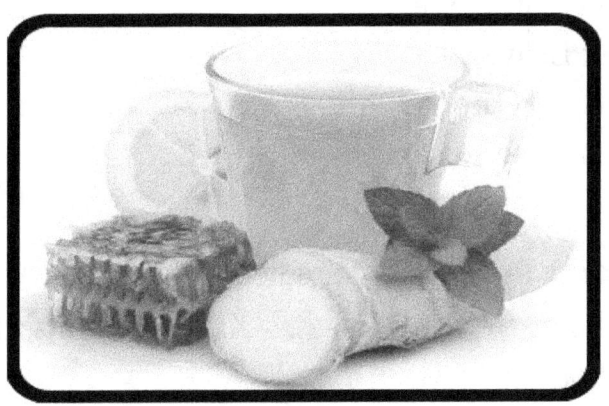

## Tea to Increase the Body's Defenses: (Very Effective):

For weeks, the natural remedy Covid Organics, an herbal drink based on the Artemisia plant, has been very popular on the African continent. Madagascar President Andry Rajoelina introduced this drug in late April. Covid Organics would fight Covid-19 and even cure COVID-19 disease. Politicians joined in the praise of this miracle remedy. Artemisinin, the active ingredient in the artemisia plant, has been used in the fight against malaria. Next Miracle tea where the ingredient of mugwort is used:

**Ingredients:**

2 or 3 slices of ginger.
2 or 3 slices of turmeric root.
2 or 3 leaves of Artemisia (this plant cures Cancer)
(Artemisia is taken for 4 days and paused for 4 days)
1 sheet of oregano.
2 branches of pure, natural Cinnamon, without additives or chemical transformation.
01 pinch of thyme
2 Mint Leaves.
1 pinch of Cardomomo.
3 branches of rosemary.

**Preparation:** Put all the ingredients in a teapot with hot water for half an hour, so that it releases all its nutrients, then take this shot throughout the day.

**Note:** Mugwort, turmeric root, and natural cinnamon can be purchased from Amazon.

# Recipes to fight Respiratory Infections, Flu, Asthma, Covid19, strengthen the Immune System.

**Syrup to increase Defenses:** This syrup has expectorant properties, garlic, onion, and ginger, each representing one of the best antibiotics out there. In addition, they have the following benefits: they help improve blood circulation, lower cholesterol, prevent chronic diseases such as arthritis, rheumatism, flu, allergies, and infections of any kind, detoxify the blood, dewormer, help to lose weight, prevents premature aging, lengthening and improving the quality of life of people.

## Recipe No. 1.
**Ingredients:**

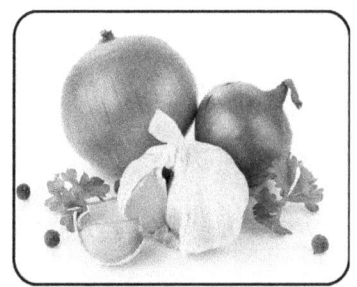

- ½ Liter of Honey
- 01 Garlic Head
- 01 purple onion
- 04 tablespoons minced ginger
- 01 Glass Bottle

**Preparation:** Peel the garlic, onion and ginger, chop it into pieces, place them inside the glass bottle, add ½ liter of honey, let it rest for 3 days. After these days strain. Store in the fridge. Adults should take 3 times a day. Children over 3 years old should take a small spoonful 2 times a day.

## *Recipe No. 2. to raise the Defenses:*
**Ingredients:**

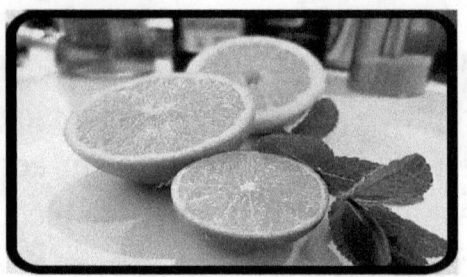

½ Kilo of Tangerines

½ lemon

250 gr. of sugar

**Preparation:** Peel the tangerines, separate into segments, remove the seeds, pour the lemon juice in a pot, and add a tablespoon of grated tangerine zest. Cook for 30 or 40 minutes, add the sugar, stirring constantly to avoid sticking. Then turn off, let stand ½ hour, pour the contents into a glass bottle. Take mid-morning daily.

## *Recipe No. 3. to raise the Defenses:*

**Ingredients:**

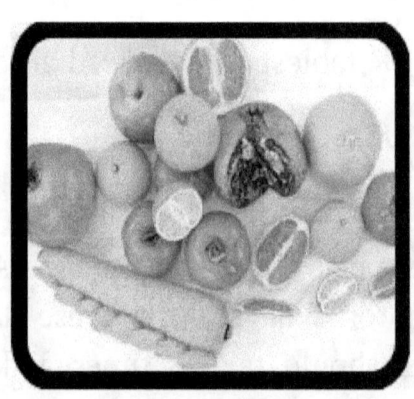

½ Liter of Water

01 Carrot

02 oranges

**Preparation:** Wash the carrots and oranges well, peel them and chop them into small pieces, add them to the blender and blend until well crushed. We serve it in a glass, add the orange juice. Take it immediately so it does not rust.

## Recipe No. 4. to strengthen the Defenses:
**Ingredients:**

- 01 Carrot, diced
- 01 Celery stalk
- 01 chopped apple
- ½ chopped cucumber
- ½ sliced beets
- ½ Bunch of Parsley

**Preparation:** Add everything to the blender, well washed and chopped into pieces. Blend, serve and drink on an empty stomach.

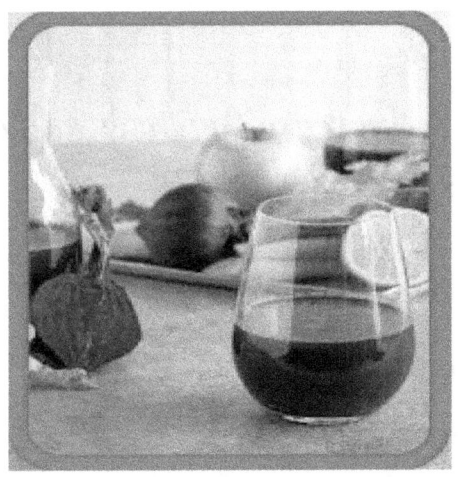

## *Recipe No. 5. to raise the Defenses:*
**Ingredients:**

- 01 Cup of Kale
- 01 Cup of Spinach
- 02 tablespoons of parsley
- 01 cucumber
- ¼ Lemon without skin (the juice)
- 01 Cup of Green Grapes or Apple

**Preparation:** Wash the vegetables very well, chop into pieces, add the lemon juice to the blender, 01 glass of water, add the grapes and the other ingredients, blend well. Take on an empty stomach every day.

## *Recipe No. 6. to increase Defenses and combat Covid19:*
**Ingredients:**

- 02 Glasses of Water
- 01 Cup of muscovado sugar
- 01 Cinnamon Stick,
- 01 teaspoon sweet cloves
- 01 teaspoon of star anise
- 01 ½ Cup of Lemon Juice
- 100 grams of ginger
- 01 glass bottle

**Preparation:** Place the 2 glasses of water, cinnamon, anise and sweet cloves to boil in a pot, once it boils, put the lemon juice and ginger, cover it, let it boil for 10 more minutes, the water should halve. Strain, once cold, pour it into the glass bottle. 01 Tablespoon is taken after breakfast and another after dinner.

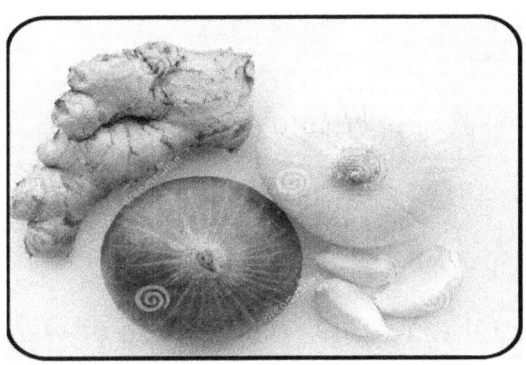

## *Recipe No. 7. Seville Lemon Water, to increase the Defenses quickly:*

**Ingredients:**

1,5 Liters of Water

08 ice cubes

02 Lemons, chopped into 4 without seeds, with skin

01 Small cup of condensed milk

01 large spoonful of sugar

**Preparation:** Of the 1.5 liters add a cup of water to the blender to liquefy the ingredients, add all the ingredients, beat well, strain and add the rest of the water in a jar, once ready add the ice. We can make this recipe three times a week and take it after breakfast.

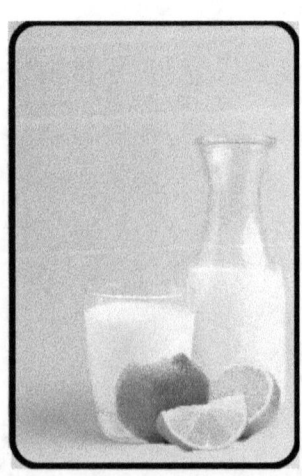

## *Recipe No. 8. To increase defenses very quickly:*

### *Ingredients:*

02 centimeters of skinless ginger

03 Lemons

½ cup of honey

01 cup of water

**Preparation:** Add all the ingredients to the blender, beat well, Strain into a jar with 1.5 liters of water. Take 01 small glass after breakfast.

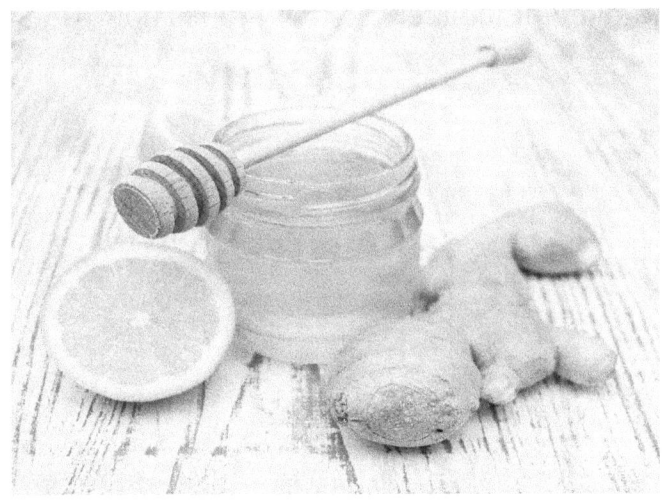

## Recipe No. 8. Shot of Ginger and Turmeric to raise the defenses:

**Ingredients:**

- 01 Lemon
- 01 Orange
- 01 Tangerine
- 03 Cm of Ginger
- 150 ml of water

**Preparation:** We remove all the shells, chop into pieces, beat in the blender, take immediately so that it does not rust, after breakfast.

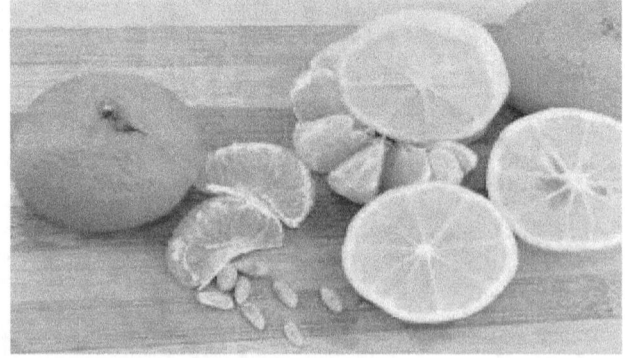

## *Vegetable Salad Recipe to Strengthen Defenses:*
### Ingredients:

01 cucumber

02 Radishes

Watercress or Spinach

02 Tomatoes

01 purple onion

03 Lemons (the juice)

Salt to taste.

### Preparation:

Wash the vegetables well, chop them into small pieces, Place them in a large container, mix all the vegetables, add the juice of the lemons, add salt to taste. This rich salad can be eaten every day, in addition to strengthening the immune system.

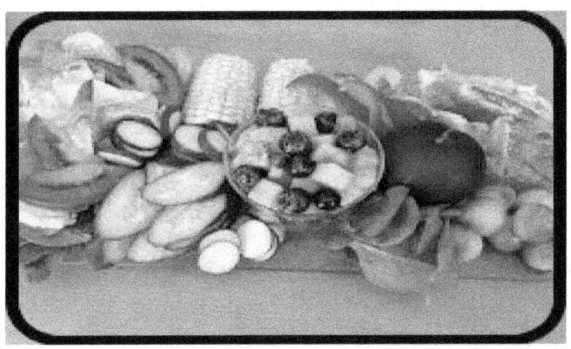

# CONCLUSION

Precisely these days we find ourselves dusting recipes and memories before the threat of the pandemic, Ecuadorians, for example, are looking for these days: ginger, lemon, star anise, cloves, turmeric, garlic, onion and honey, among other products, almost with the same concern and despair with which they look for masks, alcohol and other disinfectants, now essential to try to face the advance of the new disease.

A recipe widely used at the moment in Ecuador is the following:

Every night, lemon water with ginger, star anise, clove and turmeric should be boiled and taken hot, should be given to children and adults; it is sweetened with sugar; this drink is very good to raise the defenses. The COVID-19 has revived a series of home remedies, those transmitted from generation to generation, or used by grandmothers, which were kept filed in the drawer of memories, but that due to this disease we have seen the need to to use them again, in Ecuador and in many other countries of the world.

www.ingramcontent.com/pod-product-compliance
Lightning Source LLC
Chambersburg PA
CBHW050324220526
45465CB00005B/2127